HYPERMOBILE AND
HAPPY

Pocket Guide

Natural Healing for Hypermobility Conditions, Simplified

I0096673

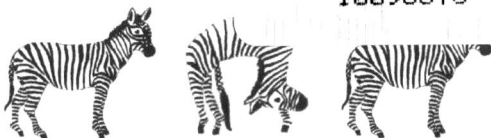

SHANNON E. GALE

Dedicated to Brandon, Edison, Kathy, Ashley, Heather, Jason, Joshu, and Paxton. In loving memory of Steven. And for hypermobile people everywhere.

For more
Hypermobile and Happy
books, merchandise, &
other offerings, scan the
QR code or visit
shannonegale.com

Hypermobile and Happy Pocket Guide: Natural Healing for Hypermobility Conditions, Simplified
Copyright © 2024 Shannon E. Gale

First Comes Love Publishing
Frankfort, Kentucky, USA

ISBN paperback: 978-1-965020-05-0
ISBN ebook: 978-1-965020-06-7

All illustrations, design, and formatting of the cover and book interior were accomplished by Shannon E. Gale.

TABLE OF CONTENTS

FEEL BETTER SOON!

Congratulations on starting your healing journey! First, read the book *Hypermobile and Happy: Naturally Heal Symptoms of Hypermobile Ehlers-Danlos Syndrome, Hypermobility Spectrum Disorders, and Many Secondary Conditions*. It will thoroughly explain each of the checklist items in this Pocket Guide.

As explained in the book, the best way to enact and maintain healing is to respond to triggers just as soon as they occur. Use this Pocket Guide to help you do that. Keep it and your most important nutritional supplements and treatment tools with you everywhere you go.

I recommend that you put a piece of clear tape over the checkboxes for the lists that you need to use. When you get triggered, use a fine-tip dry-erase marker on the tape to check each item as you complete it. Then, once the symptom flare has passed, erase your marks from the tape so that the book is ready to use when you need it again.

From time to time, re-read the portions of the book that you need the most. Without the book's explanations, the Pocket Guide's checklist items could easily be misunderstood or confusing.

If you get triggered, try to remain calm. Don't get stressed out or worried. Trust in your ability to take care of yourself, and have faith that this shall pass and you will feel better soon!

Joint Instability & Pain

RECOGNIZE WHEN A JOINT IS THREATENED OR HYPEREXTENDED

Ask your doctor before trying anything new.

- ☐ The joint hurts.
- ☐ Body parts near the joint hurt —sharp stabbing, dull ache, throbbing.
- ☐ Muscle cramps or spasms near the joint.
- ☐ The joint locks up.
- ☐ Tingling or numbness in the joint or another body part.
- ☐ Weakness or trembling.
- ☐ Breathlessness or fatigue.
- ☐ Your body looks funny (to you or someone else).

AVOID JOINT INJURY

- ☐ Stop purposefully or accidentally stretching/hyperextending.
- ☐ Change position every 2 minutes.
- ☐ Analyze all of your movement patterns throughout the day and work to improve them.
- ☐ Improve posture from head to foot.
- ☐ Use braces, ring splints, SI belts (for the sacroiliac joints of the hips), etc. as needed for weak joints.
- ☐ Use tools that make the job easier.
- ☐ Opt for clothing with zippers rather than snaps and buttons.
- ☐ Do Strength Training very carefully.
- ☐ Cross train.
- ☐ Sleep toes and nose to the ceiling.
- ☐ In the car and other places where you must sit still, use small pillows or other tools to support the body.
- ☐ Follow the Cusack Protocol of supplements.
- ☐ Eliminate infections.

- ☐ Be more cautious when other symptoms flare up due to triggers.
- ☐ Be more cautious at times of changing hormone levels.
- ☐ Follow a "Life Hacks" social media group.
- ☐ Stand up for yourself.

RECOVER FROM JOINT INJURY

- ☐ Use ice to prevent and reduce inflammation.
- ☐ Apply comfrey to the skin at the site of the injury.
- ☐ Apply heat to relax muscles.
- ☐ Massage.
- ☐ Keep moving, but do not move in ways that hurt.
- ☐ Use KT Tape, a brace, splint, or a sling to stabilize the affected joint.
- ☐ Use Near-Infrared and Red Light Therapy to heal injuries and tighten skin.

- ☐ Follow the Pilates videos by Jeannie di Bon or another hypermobility movement specialist.

- ☐ Use Earthing Therapy Patches applied to the affected area.

- ☐ Apply magnesium oil to the skin where muscles are tight.

- ☐ Meditate.

- ☐ Find good, reliable professionals who are familiar with hEDS and HSD.

REDUCE THE UNPLEASANT EFFECTS
OF ALLERGY/MCAS/MCS

Ask your doctor before trying anything new.

☐ Figure out what environmental components, household chemicals, and foods you are sensitive to.

☐ Avoid anything you are allergic or sensitive to.

☐ Choose organic, all-natural, fragrance-free toiletries, and cleaning products.

☐ Eat only organic, all-natural foods.

☐ Avoid toxic chemicals, even if they are not harmful in small doses to most people.

☐ Avoid having anything implanted into your body.

☐ Avoid Electromagnetic Frequency Radiation (EMFs).

☐ Keep the air in your home clean.

- Keep your vehicle scent-free.
- Request accommodations at your workplace, school, and church.

CALM YOUR SYSTEM EVERY DAY TO REDUCE SENSITIVITY TO FOOD, CHEMICALS, STRESS, & SENSORY INPUTS

- Prevent your joints from hyperextending.
- Follow a daily rhythm that works for you.
- Follow a weekly rhythm.
- Follow a yearly rhythm that is inspired by the seasons.
- Avoid any foods and environmental substances that trigger you.
- Eat warm, soft foods, and drink warm beverages.
- Limit foods like peppers, onions, and garlic that are known to excite the immune system.
- Do not eat leftovers or overripe foods.

- [ ] Take DAO right before eating and sleeping.
- [ ] Get massages or give them to yourself.
- [ ] Tap the thymus.
- [ ] Take warm baths.
- [ ] Feel gratitude.
- [ ] Spend time in nature.
- [ ] Snuggle and cuddle with someone you care about or a pet.
- [ ] Keep warm.
- [ ] Avoid electronics.
- [ ] Play.
- [ ] Sing.
- [ ] Listen to music, and if you feel like it, dance like no one is watching.
- [ ] Don't rush.
- [ ] Eliminate infections.
- [ ] Take quercetin or berberine to stabilize mast cells.
- [ ] Eat culinary and wildgrown herbs.
- [ ] Drink AllergEase Tea daily.

- [ ] Detox your body and your lifestyle.
- [ ] Take trace minerals.
- [ ] Get auricular acupuncture.

TAKE PREVENTATIVE MEASURES FOR RISKY SITUATIONS WHEN YOU ANTICIPATE BEING EXPOSED TO ENVIRONMENTAL ALLERGENS

- [ ] Take supplements.
- [ ] One baby aspirin.
- [ ] Grape Juice or tart cherry juice.
- [ ] Vitamin C with bioflavonoids or ascorbic acid.
- [ ] Magnesium.
- [ ] Homeopathic Ignatia amara.
- [ ] Astragalus.
- [ ] Milk thistle.
- [ ] Methylfolate and Methylcolbalmin.
- [ ] Bioplasma cell salts.
- [ ] DAO
- [ ] Rebound or do Lymph Drainage Massage.
- [ ] Wear a personal ionizer.

- [ ] Wear a mask when you do not have a personal ionizer.

- [ ] Wrap hair or wear a hood or hat so that your hair won't absorb scent, and bring a change of clothes.

- [ ] Apply refined shea butter on any exposed skin to protect against getting allergens on the skin.

- [ ] Wear sunglasses to filter out too-bright or flickering lights.

- [ ] Wear specialty ear plugs to filter out background noise.

PREVENT AND REDUCE SYMPTOMS OF ALLERGY/MCAS/MCS AFTER EXPOSURES

- [ ] Wipe skin down with a wet cloth immediately after exposure.

- [ ] Take Homeopathic Remedies as needed.

  - [ ] Overexertion and physical or emotional trauma: *Arnica Montana*.

  - [ ] Difficulty breathing and fatigue: *Arsenicum album*.

- [ ] Inflamed mucous membranes, sore throat, and sinus congestion: *Belladonna.*

- [ ] Body aches and exhaustion: *Chamomilla.*

- [ ] Stiff neck and tension headache: *Gelsemium.*

- [ ] Swelling in face, sneezing, coughing: *Histaminum hydrochloricum.*

- [ ] Allergic reaction initial stage and anxiety: *Ignatia amara.*

- [ ] Muscle tension and anxiety: *Magnesium phosphorica.*

- [ ] Sores in mouth: *Mercurius solubus.*

- [ ] Nausea and Insomnia caused by worry: *Nux vomica.*

- [ ] Exposure to petroleum products such as synthetic fragrances and gasoline: *Petroleum.*

- [ ] Cough and chest congestion: *Phosphorous.*

- [ ] Sinus pressure and sneezing: *Pulsatilla.*

- [ ] Hopelessness, feeling overwhelmed, and menstrual cramps: *Sepia.*

- [ ] Deep-seated fear: *Stramonium.*

- [ ] Take supplements.
    - [ ] Activated charcoal.
    - [ ] Magnesium malate.
    - [ ] DAO.
    - [ ] B vitamins.
    - [ ] Vitamin C (ascorbic acid).
    - [ ] Stinging nettle.
    - [ ] Milk thistle.
    - [ ] Methylfolate and methylcobalamin simultaneously.
    - [ ] Salty and fatty foods.
    - [ ] Water.
    - [ ] Baking soda.
    - [ ] Grape juice or tart cherry juice.
    - [ ] Electrolytes.
    - [ ] Alka Seltzer Gold.
    - [ ] Multivitamins.
    - [ ] TRS (Toxin and Contaminant Removal System) by Coseva.
    - [ ] Collagen peptides.
    - [ ] Single baby aspirin every 12 hours.
    - [ ] Topical magnesium

PREVENT CEREBELLAR DISORDERS FOLLOWING TRIGGER EXPOSURE

Ask your doctor before trying anything new.

☐ Use oxygen therapy.

☐ Eat basil, oregano, parsley, and/or turmeric.

☐ Take acetylcholine, methylfolate, methylcolbalamin, thiamine, and B6.

COPE WITH CEREBELLAR ATAXIA CLUMSINESS

☐ Avoid dangerous cooking.

☐ Ask family members or friends to help with risky tasks.

☐ Avoid driving vehicles while experiencing Ataxia.

☐ Do not use exercise equipment but instead move slowly and hold onto something for balance when you exercise.

☐ Use braces, canes, and other tools to help protect your joints.

☐ Meditate with deep breathing and become as calm as possible.

REDUCE DIGESTIVE SYSTEM PROBLEMS

Ask your doctor before trying anything new.

- ☐ Do elimination diets and keep diaries to figure out what you are sensitive to, and then avoid those things no matter what.

- ☐ Avoid your food and environmental allergens.

- ☐ Live a wholesome lifestyle.

- ☐ Take probiotics and eat prebiotic foods.

- ☐ Eat whole foods as much as possible.

- ☐ Choose organic foods.

- ☐ Prepare, store, and serve your food using nontoxic dishes, pots, pans, and utensils.

- ☐ Sit up straight, especially when you eat and for 3 hours afterward.

- ☐ Don't wear clothes that are tight around the abdomen.

- Chew your food thoroughly.
- Pay attention to your cravings.
- Eat porridge.
- Limit foods that are likely to upset the stomach or cause inflammation.
- Drink lots of water and healthy drinks.
- Filter your water to remove all contaminants.
- Drink a glass of water half an hour before a meal, but drink very little with your meal.
- Bless your food.
- Eat early in the day.
- Use homeopathic remedies.
- Drink a small dose of baking soda in water.
- Use Earthing Therapy Patches on your stomach.
- Stimulate the Vagus Nerve.
- Protect your cervical spine.
- Get Chiropractic or Osteopathic care.
- Take trace minerals.

- [ ] Try taking DAO 15 minutes before meals.
- [ ] Try eating standing up.

Eye Strain

PREVENT AND RECOVER FROM EYE STRAIN

Ask your doctor before trying anything new.

- ☐ Avoid looking at screens.
- ☐ Take frequent breaks when looking at screens or reading books.
- ☐ Exercise the eyes with the Bates Method.
- ☐ Go without sunglasses.

MENSTRUATION

Ask your doctor before trying anything new.

- ☐ Use all-natural, organic products.
- ☐ Do abdominal self-massage.
- ☐ Anticipate menstruation by using a Saliva Ovulation Microscope.
- ☐ Use extra caution to protect joints and avoid triggers during menstruation or ovulation, whichever hormone surge is most likely to make you more sensitive.

STRATEGIES FOR CONTRACEPTION

- ☐ Get to know your own body's cycles.
- ☐ Ask your doctor or midwife for guidance.

FERTILITY BOOSTING IDEAS

- ☐ Heal your symptoms of hEDS/HSD and secondary conditions.
- ☐ Read *It Starts with the Egg*.
- ☐ Get Chiropractic or Osteopathic care.
- ☐ Get Acupuncture and Traditional Chinese Medicine treatment.
- ☐ Eliminate silent infections.
- ☐ Baby Dance on the few days leading up to ovulation.
- ☐ Reduce stress.
- ☐ Get a professional Mayan Abdominal Massage.

REDUCE HYPEREMESIS GRAVIDARUM NAUSEA

- ☐ Keep the nausea minimized as much as possible.
- ☐ Keep your MCAS under control.

- [ ] Take organic liquid chlorophyll.

- [ ] Use Homeopathic Remedies such as *Nux vomica*.

- [ ] If drinking liquids exacerbates your nausea, chew pellet ice instead.

- [ ] When nausea is severe, drink one fountain soda and then eat a high fat, high protein meal.

- [ ] Eat a small candy to prepare for eating a meal.

- [ ] Wear a Sea Band wrist acupressure band on one wrist and an electric shock wristband on the other wrist.

- [ ] Protect the joints.

- [ ] Take Papaya Enzyme with meals.

- [ ] Chew gum after a meal.

- [ ] Reconsider taking vitamins.

- [ ] Eat high-protein snacks.

- [ ] Massage acupressure points.

- [ ] Use disposable dishes and utensils

COPING STRATEGIES FOR SUBCHORIONIC HEMATOMA

- ☐ Follow your doctor's orders.
- ☐ Rest in bed.
- ☐ Pray.

TREAT PLANTAR FASCIITIS

Ask your doctor before trying anything new.

- ☐ Roll balls under your feet.
- ☐ Massage the foot and leg.
- ☐ Avoid hyperextending the knees.
- ☐ Keep the muscles of the lower leg balanced between the front (shin) and back (calf).
- ☐ Elongate the muscles of the back of the legs.
- ☐ Do not point the toes when it is not necessary.
- ☐ Give yourself foot baths.
- ☐ Moisturize with organic oils.
- ☐ Use Earthing Therapy Patches on your feet.
- ☐ Wear barefoot/minimalist shoes.

HEAL BUNIONS WITHOUT SURGERY

- ☐ Do foot yoga.
- ☐ Stand with proper posture.
- ☐ Balance the muscles of the lower leg.
- ☐ Walk barefoot on uneven ground.
- ☐ Wear barefoot/minimalist shoes.
- ☐ Make sure your socks and slippers are not tight.
- ☐ Apply magnesium oil.
- ☐ Wear toe separators.

HEAL FLAT FEET

- ☐ Do *tendus*.
- ☐ Do *dégagés* and *grand battements*.
- ☐ Do *relevés*.
- ☐ Do not wear arch supports.

EASE GROWING PAINS

Ask your doctor before trying anything new.

- [ ] Apply ice.
- [ ] Apply heat.
- [ ] Massage.
- [ ] Apply comfrey oil.
- [ ] Apply magnesium oil.
- [ ] Offer Arnica montana.
- [ ] See an Osteopath.
- [ ] Treat possible joint injuries.
- [ ] Get Physical Therapy.

Hand Pain

REDUCE HAND PAIN

Ask your doctor before trying anything new.

- ☐ Do Earthing daily.
- ☐ Wear ring splints.
- ☐ Do Rice Bucket Exercises.
- ☐ Do Lymph Drainage Massage.
- ☐ Apply comfrey oil.

HEAL DUPUYTREN'S CONTRACTURE

- ☐ Stretch the fingers back (but not too far) and hold for 30 seconds.
- ☐ Use the other thumb to massage the palm of your hand where the bumps or indentations are, pressing toward the heart for 30 seconds.

☐ Apply heat and magnesium oil.

☐ Apply comfrey oil.

PREVENT AND TREAT KNEE PAIN

Ask your doctor before trying anything new.

- ☐ Stand with correct posture.
- ☐ Do the seated knee strengthening exercise.
- ☐ Do Range of Motion exercises for the hips and ankles.
- ☐ Get help from a Physical Therapist.

Lymph Congestion

IMPROVE LYMPH FLOW

Ask your doctor before trying anything new.

- ☐ Get a Lymph Drainage Massage.
- ☐ Rebound gently on a trampoline.
- ☐ Dry brush before bathing.
- ☐ Do Abhyanga Oil Massage.
- ☐ Go for long walks.
- ☐ Vibrate the entire body.
- ☐ Do or receive Gua Sha scraping.
- ☐ Take an herbal blend for lymph support.
- ☐ Drink a lot of water.

Migraine

PREVENT MIGRAINE ATTACKS

Ask your doctor before trying anything new.

- ☐ Figure out your triggers and avoid them.
- ☐ Minimize the potency of your triggers if you can't avoid them completely.
- ☐ Keep your Migraine treatments ready and easily accessible.
- ☐ Avoid caffeine and alcohol.
- ☐ Pray.

RECOGNIZE MIGRAINE ATTACKS

- ☐ Ask others to help by telling you if they see signs that you have been triggered.
- ☐ Notice if others are doing annoying things.
- ☐ Look in the mirror from time to time.

- [ ] Notice what difficulties you are having.

- [ ] Notice if the environment is providing too much sensation.

- [ ] Notice if your emotional state has changed.

- [ ] Correlate returning or worsening symptoms with the trigger.

PREVENT MIGRAINE ATTACKS AFTER BEING TRIGGERED

- [ ] Drink grapefruit juice.

- [ ] Take Homeopathic Remedies.

- [ ] Take one baby aspirin.

- [ ] Drink ¼ teaspoon baking soda in 2 ounces water.

- [ ] Breathe oxygen.

- [ ] Take riboflavin, B12, and folate.

- [ ] Do The Basic Exercise.

- [ ] Do the Red Ball Exercises.

- ☐ Lie down in the dark for an hour.
- ☐ Do Earthing.

REDUCE MIGRAINE ATTACK DEVELOPMENT

- ☐ Take electrolytes.
- ☐ Eat fatty, salty foods.
- ☐ Get shoulder and back massage.
- ☐ Take it easy.
- ☐ Continue Earthing.
- ☐ Use an herb that is known to reduce pain, such as peppermint or chamomile.
- ☐ If the headache pain is very severe, take an adult dose of aspirin.

REDUCE THE SEVERITY OF A MIGRAINE ATTACK

- ☐ Take a hot shower.
- ☐ Use hydrotherapy.
- ☐ Take one baby aspirin.
- ☐ Drink more electrolytes.
- ☐ Eat chocolate.
- ☐ Stay relaxed in the dark.
- ☐ Apply heat or cold.
- ☐ Use a Zok device in the ear.
- ☐ Do gua sha scraping of the neck.
- ☐ Do self-acupressure.
- ☐ Do self-Reiki.
- ☐ Use a Near Infrared and Red Light Therapy box.
- ☐ Get fresh air.
- ☐ Endeavor to keep good posture.
- ☐ Take a nap.

Motion Sickness

CURE MOTION SICKNESS

Ask your doctor before trying anything new.

- [ ] Keep your eyes on the road or water in front of you.
- [ ] Wear Motion Sickness Glasses.
- [ ] Wear Sea Bands.
- [ ] Wear an electric shock bracelet.
- [ ] Sit in a supported position.
- [ ] Sleep.
- [ ] Drive.
- [ ] Put the breeze in your face.
- [ ] Use Homeopathic Remedies such as *Nux vomica*, *Tabacum*, *Ipecacuanha*, and *Cocculus indicus*.
- [ ] Eat peppermint candy.

TOOTH AND GUM CARE

Ask your doctor before trying anything new.

- ☐ Brush your teeth twice per day.
- ☐ Use a Bass toothbrush.
- ☐ Use remineralizing tooth powder.
- ☐ Brush the front top of the tongue.
- ☐ Floss your teeth daily.
- ☐ Do oil pulling occasionally and as needed.
- ☐ Do not use mouthwash on a regular basis.
- ☐ Follow the diet in *Cure Tooth Decay*.
- ☐ Moisturize lips with organic refined shea butter.
- ☐ Do not get amalgam fillings.

CREATE HEALTHY MOUTH POSTURE

- ☐ Practice mewing.
- ☐ Chew a lot.
- ☐ Do Buteyko Mouth Taping during sleep.
- ☐ Eliminate tongue and buccal ties.
- ☐ Keep your "resting bliss face" on.
- ☐ Relieve hypertonicity in jaw muscles.
- ☐ Use good sitting posture at the dining table.

COMPENSATE FOR MTHFR

Ask your doctor before trying anything new.

- ☐ Get medical help and study Dr. Lynch's recommendations.
- ☐ Detox your lifestyle.
- ☐ Detox your body.
- ☐ Consider chelating.

Neck Pain

PREVENT AND TREAT NECK PAIN

Ask your doctor before trying anything new.

- ☐ Maintain correct head posture.
- ☐ If your neck gets tired, lie down to rest.
- ☐ Do The Basic Exercise.
- ☐ Maintain correct tongue posture.
- ☐ Do Range of Motion exercises very slowly.
- ☐ Do Red Ball Exercises.
- ☐ When lying down, use a rolled-up towel or specialty pillow to support the curve of the neck.
- ☐ Do the suboccipital muscle stretch.
- ☐ Do neck stretches.
- ☐ Use heat.
- ☐ Massage.
- ☐ Do Myofascial Release Massage.

- ☐ Cope with stress by keeping good posture.
- ☐ Apply comfrey oil.
- ☐ Use Homeopathic Remedies.
- ☐ Treat any nerve damage.
- ☐ Do advanced neck strengthening exercises.

PREVENT AND REVERSE
OSTEOPENIA AND OSTEOPOROSIS

Ask your doctor before trying anything new.

- ☐ Jump.

- ☐ Do resistance training.

- ☐ Take collagen peptides.

- ☐ Take vitamins and minerals.

- ☐ Get sunlight.

- ☐ Maintain a healthy gut microbiome by taking *L-rhamnosus GG*.

- ☐ Reduce inflammation.

TREAT PELVIS COMPLAINTS

Ask your doctor before trying anything new.

☐ Get pelvic specialty Physical Therapy.

☐ Avoid harming your joints further.

☐ Try some of the go-to maneuvers for the pelvis.

TREAT AND COPE WITH PERIPHERAL NEUROPATHY

Ask your doctor before trying anything new.

- ☐ Relieve pressure on the site of the injury.

- ☐ Prevent yourself from scratching.

- ☐ Apply evening primrose oil to the skin at the site of the injury.

- ☐ Take acetylcholine, methylfolate, methylcolbalamin, thiamine, and B6.

- ☐ Apply ice to the location of the symptom.

- ☐ Apply magnesium oil to the location of the symptom.

- ☐ Apply heat to the location of the injury.

- ☐ Drink grape juice.

- ☐ Eat culinary herbs that support nerve health.

- ☐ Use Homeopathic Remedies.

- Do light exercise that does not endanger the site of the injury but uses the sites of symptoms.

- Do Earthing.

- Use Near Infrared and Red Light Therapy.

- Get Reiki.

- Avoid any neurotoxic medications, chemicals, or foods.

- Pray, use Affirmations, and try Forest Bathing.

PREVENT POTS EPISODES

Ask your doctor before trying anything new.

- ☐ Take electrolytes daily.
- ☐ Get out of bed slowly.
- ☐ Stand up slowly.
- ☐ Don't bend over.
- ☐ Avoid climbing hills or stairs.
- ☐ Avoid standing still.
- ☐ Avoid stressful situations.
- ☐ Wear compression socks or stockings.
- ☐ Avoid caffeine.
- ☐ Do not overeat.
- ☐ Drink plenty of water and eat sufficient salt.
- ☐ Maintain proper head and neck posture.
- ☐ Do not hyperextend your knees.

- ☐ Follow the Cusack Protocol.
- ☐ Exercise.
- ☐ Build postural orthostatic tolerance.
- ☐ Take extra precautions when you are having your menstrual period.

RECOVER QUICKLY FROM POTS EPISODES

- ☐ Pay attention to POTS warning signs.
- ☐ Drink electrolytes.
- ☐ Lie down with feet up.
- ☐ Put feet and lower legs in cold water.
- ☐ Drink caffeine.
- ☐ Do the Valsalva Maneuver or cough.

Rib Cage Pain

RETURN STRENGTH AND FLEXIBILITY TO THE RIB CAGE TO REDUCE PAIN

Ask your doctor before trying anything new.

- ☐ Do Jeannie di Bon's Pilates exercises.
- ☐ Apply heat to the area.
- ☐ Gently massage the entire rib cage.
- ☐ Release the fascia of the rib cage.
- ☐ Pop the rib(s) back into position, if necessary.
- ☐ Do pull overs and rows.
- ☐ Exercise the serratus anterior muscles.
- ☐ Apply comfrey oil.
- ☐ Do the Cusack Protocol.
- ☐ Keep awareness of the injured area.
- ☐ Sleep in safe, supported positions.

SWIM TO TREAT SCOLIOSIS

Ask your doctor before trying anything new.

- Stay upright in the pool if you have POTS, doing aerobics or treading water.

- Avoid or protect against chlorine if you have MCAS.

- Alternate different swim strokes and activities.

- Drink water with electrolytes before swimming.

- Practice deep breathing before beginning a swimming routine.

- Rinse and moisturize after swimming.

- Massage after swimming.

- Do Myofascial Release Massage once you have built up strength.

PREVENT SKIN CONDITIONS

Ask your doctor before trying anything new.

- ☐ Keep the skin clean.
- ☐ Wash your face with the Oil Cleansing Method.
- ☐ Use only gentle, all-natural moisturizers.
- ☐ Use only all-natural makeup or none at all.
- ☐ Prevent body acne by taking baths with Epsom salts.
- ☐ Take Vitamin C.
- ☐ Do not wear sunglasses all of the time.
- ☐ Eat watermelon when you are going to be in the sun.

TREAT SHOULDER PAIN

Ask your doctor before trying anything new.

- [ ] Do not move out of the appropriate range of motion.
- [ ] Sleep on your back with pillow support.
- [ ] Apply ice.
- [ ] Get massage.
- [ ] Get Physical Therapy.
- [ ] Get Myofascial Release Massage.
- [ ] Apply heat.
- [ ] Get Reiki.

REDUCE SINUS CONGESTION

Ask your doctor before trying anything new.

- [ ] Do Lymph Drainage Massage of the face and neck.
- [ ] Use Homeopathic Remedies *Pulsatilla* and *Phosphorus*.
- [ ] Spend as much time outside as possible.
- [ ] Use peppermint or other herbal teas.
- [ ] Use pseudoephedrine or ephedra.
- [ ] Breathe steam.
- [ ] Use cotton handkerchiefs.
- [ ] Use a Neti Pot.

Thoracic Outlet Syndrome

TREAT THORACIC OUTLET SYNDROME

Ask your doctor before trying anything new.

- ☐ Correct your back and shoulder posture.
- ☐ Get an adjustment from a Chiropractor or Osteopath.
- ☐ Stretch out your chest.
- ☐ Stretch the pectoralis muscles.
- ☐ Do a Kneeling Thoracic Stretch.
- ☐ Strengthen your back by lifting weights.
- ☐ Do Shoulder External Rotation exercises.
- ☐ Breathe deeply into your belly and keep the ribs mobile.
- ☐ Do self-massage.
- ☐ Do Myofascial Release Massage.

Heal Symptoms of TMJ

Ask your doctor before trying anything new.

- [ ] Meditate to relax the muscles of the face.
- [ ] Eat soft foods.
- [ ] Don't move the jaw in ways that hurt.
- [ ] Improve posture.
- [ ] Use heat and/or ice.
- [ ] Seek help from a professional therapist.
- [ ] Get Craniosacral Therapy, Osteopathy, or Chiropractic care.
- [ ] Massage.
- [ ] Do Myofascial Release Massage.
- [ ] Exercise and listen to music.
- [ ] Treat Trigeminal Neuralgia, if present.

www.ingramcontent.com/pod-product-compliance
Lightning Source LLC
Chambersburg PA
CBHW052026030426

42335CB00026B/3299